Calculations for Nurses

*Related Faber titles*

THE NURSES' DICTIONARY 30th Edition
**Christine Brooker**

NEW FABER ANATOMICAL ATLAS
**Anne Roberts and Audrey Besterman**

PRINCIPAL DRUGS 9th Edition
**S. J. Hopkins**

SPECIAL TESTS 13th Edition
**D. M. D. Evans**

# Calculations for Nurses

G. W. Watchorn, MPS
*Formerly Area Pharmaceutical Officer,*
*Greenwich and Bexley Area Health Authority*

*Revised by*
Jill Gregson
*Nurse Tutor,*
*St Mary's Hospital School of Nursing, London*

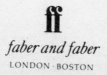

*faber and faber*
LONDON · BOSTON

First published as *Medical Calculations for Nurses* in 1973
by Faber and Faber Ltd
3 Queen Square London WC1
Reprinted 1975
Second edition 1976, reprinted 1978 and 1982
Third edition 1989

Photoset by Parker Typesetting Service Leicester
Printed in Great Britain by
Richard Clay Ltd Bungay Suffolk
All rights reserved

© G. W. Watchorn, 1973, 1976
New material © Jill Gregson, 1989

A CIP record for this book is available from the British Library

ISBN 0-571-14077-7

# Contents

# Preface to Third Edition

Since this book was first produced, the nurse's need for numeracy skills has been demonstrated by research (S. Pirie,* 1987). It is clear that this little book could assist those in training to see the relevance of these skills to their everyday work.

Several alterations have been made throughout the text, to bring examples up to date, and the addition of exercises at the end of each chapter helps the reader to check his or her understanding.

Jill Gregson 1988

## ACKNOWLEDGEMENT

I am grateful to the Department of Health for permission to reproduce Table 4, *Recommended daily intakes of energy and nutrients for the UK*, 1979 (Department of Health).

* S. Pirie (1987) *Nurses and Mathematics* RCN, London.

# Chapter One

## The Metric System

The United Kingdom, like many other countries of the world, has been using the metric system for a number of measurements in clinical and pharmaceutical practice for many years. Some countries however (including the UK) have in the past clung to units which were peculiar to that country but meant little to anyone else.

It became necessary therefore to establish a uniform system which everybody could understand. In 1960 the General Conference of Weights and Measures, meeting in Paris, suggested that the Système International d'Unités, or SI units, should be adopted throughout the world, and there has been a gradual move in that direction since that date. The British government confirmed its intentions to change any remaining units to SI by the end of 1975.

### SI UNITS

The system is based on the metric system and is designed to limit the unit used for any physical quantity to one kind only. It is used by all disciplines including not only nurses but doctors, pharmacists, laboratory technicians and hospital engineers – so the units used will range from steam pressure units to units for blood plasma analyses. There are seven so-called *base units* which are listed in the following table.

Note that each has its own symbol, which may or may not be a capital letter. *This is important.*

**Base units**

| Physical quantity | Name of SI unit | Symbol of SI unit |
|---|---|---|
| Length | metre | m |
| Mass | kilogram | kg |
| Time | second | s |
| Electric current | ampere | A |
| Thermodynamic temperature | kelvin | K |
| Luminous intensity | candela | cd |
| Amount of substance | mole | mol |

Length, time, mass (i.e. weight) and amount of substance (mole) are the ones that a nurse is likely to be involved in.

**Derived units**

Derived units are a combination of base units, and again the symbols are important. While the joule (J) and pascal (Pa) are the only two derived units of direct concern to the nurse, the table below is included to illustrate the wide application of the system.

| Quantity | Name of SI unit | Symbol | Expression in terms of SI base units or derived units |
| --- | --- | --- | --- |
| Force | newton | N | $1\,N = 1\,kg\,m/s^2$ |
| Work, energy, quantity of heat | joule | J | $1\,J = 1\,N\,m$ |
| Power | watt | W | $1\,W = 1\,J/s$ |
| Pressure | pascal | Pa | $1\,Pa = 1\,N/m^2$ $= 1\,kg/m\,s^2$ |
| Frequency | hertz | Hz | $1\,Hz = 1/s$ |
| Quantity of electricity | coulomb | C | $1\,C = 1\,A\,s$ |
| Electric potential, potential difference, tension, electromotive force | volt | V | $1\,V = 1\,W/A$ |
| Electric resistance | ohm | Ω | $1\,\Omega = 1\,V/a$ |
| Flux of magnetic induction, magnetic flux | weber | Wb | $1\,Wb = 1\,V\,s$ |
| Induction | henry | H | $1\,H = 1\,V\,s/A$ |

| Quantity | Name of SI unit | Symbol | Expression in terms of SI base units or derived units |
|---|---|---|---|
| Magnetic flux density, magnetic induction | tesla | T | $1\ T = 1\ Wb/m^2$ |
| Electric capacitance | farad | F | $1\ F = 1\ A\ s/V$ |

## Multiples of SI units and practical applications

Multiples are formed with the use of prefixes and indices, and there are specific rules as to their use and the way they are written. They will be found mainly in laboratory reports. The numbers used in these reports are such that many noughts are involved, which can easily lead to mistakes if the rules are not strictly adhered to. For example, the difference between a capital M for $10^6$ and a small m for $10^{-3}$ is *one thousand million*.

## Indices

As a help to those who are not familiar with the use of indices, you can remember best by observing that:

(*a*) For numbers *above* one, the index number is *the same* as the number of noughts, e.g. one million = 1000 000 = $10^6$, i.e. six noughts.

(*b*) For numbers *below* one, the index figure has a minus sign and is *one more than* the number of noughts to the right of the decimal point, e.g. 1 microgram ($\mu$g) could be written 0·000 001 gram = $10^{-6}$ g, and 1/100 = 0·01 = $10^{-2}$.

Note that a nought is always placed *in front of the decimal point* in instances of quantities less than one.

Note also that there are no commas between the noughts, but the noughts are grouped in threes with a space between them. *Commas have no place in the SI system.*

A further point to note is that units remain unaltered in the plural, that is *there are no added s's.* One milligram is written 1 mg and ten milligrams is written 10 mg (*not* 10 mgs).

In the case of the *microgram*, the rules say that when typing and if the typewriter is fitted with the correct key, the sign $\mu$g may be used. To avoid confusion, it is recommended that no attempt should be made to abbreviate when prescriptions are handwritten, and that the word microgram be written out in full every time.

Indices such as, for example, $10^6$ for a megaunit of penicillin, should *never* be used for writing prescriptions.

## Time

Although the standard unit for time is the second, there are occasions in medicine when a *24 hour specimen* is collected. The recognized symbol for day is 'd', but as this could be interpreted as representing daylight hours only the term 24 hours is still used. A faecal excretion report would be expressed as so many grams per 24 hours or g/24 hours.

## Volume measurements and concentrations

To be consistent with the system, the standard unit for volume would be the cubic metre, but as this is so enormous for everyday use the *litre* is used as the standard for liquid volumes, and all concentrations are quoted with reference to the litre, either as mass concentration which is *weight in volume*, e.g. grams per litre, or as *molar concentration* (see page 24).

5

The changeover from the imperial system of grains and drachms of the apothecaries' scale, and ounces and pounds of the avoirdupois system, was done over a number of years in three stages. The first change concerned the pharmaceutical industry. A high proportion of the British industry's output is exported, and most of the countries to which the products were sent used the metric system for their everyday transactions. For reasons of economy they therefore decided to market all their output in metric sizes. Hospital pharmacists in Britain were thus required to order, for example, not 4 lb of bicarbonate of soda but 2 kilograms (kg).

The next stage involved the nurse. All single-dose medications such as injections and tablets were reformulated by the manufacturers to metric doses. This meant, for instance, that the common 5 grain aspirin became 300 milligrams (mg), and what used to be known as a ¼ grain morphia injection changed to 15 milligrams.

Finally, with the publication of the 1968 British National Formulary (BNF), all fluid preparations, such as mixtures or elixirs, had their formulae changed so that the dose was always a standard 5 millilitre (ml) spoonful or multiples of the same. Pharmacists are obliged to issue with these preparations a plastic spoon of exactly 5 ml capacity. Modern medicines are potent preparations and it is *essential* that the patient receives the correct dose, hence the use of this standard spoon rather than the many varieties and sizes of domestic spoons.

We shall now examine the metric system in more detail and compare it with the old method. All means of measuring have to start with a standard unit. In the imperial and avoirdupois systems, no longer used for medicines but still used to measure household products in the United Kingdom, the unit common to both systems is the ounce. Reference to the tables below shows that the multiples above and below the ounce are widely varying numbers.

## Apothecaries' fluid measure

$$60 \text{ minims (drops)} = 1 \text{ drachm}$$
$$8 \text{ drachms} \quad = 1 \text{ ounce}$$
$$20 \text{ ounces} \quad = 1 \text{ pint}$$
Multiples 60, 8, 20

## Avoirdupois weights

$$437\frac{1}{2} \text{ grains} = 1 \text{ ounce}$$
$$16 \text{ ounces} = 1 \text{ pound}$$
$$14 \text{ pounds} = 1 \text{ stone}$$
Multiples $437\frac{1}{2}$, 16, 14

In the metric system, whether you are measuring by weight or by volume, this number *without exception* is always 10.

## METRIC WEIGHTS

## Base unit for weight: kilogram (kg)

$$10 \text{ milligrams} = 1 \text{ centigram}$$
$$10 \text{ centigrams} = 1 \text{ decigram}$$
$$10 \text{ decigrams} = 1 \text{ gram}$$
$$10 \text{ grams} \quad = 1 \text{ decagram}$$
$$10 \text{ decagrams} = 1 \text{ hectogram}$$
$$10 \text{ hectograms} = 1 \text{ kilogram}$$

In practice, we only use three of these stages, the milligram, the gram and the kilogram.

In addition one other weight is used when only very small doses are required. This is the microgram ($\mu$g), which is 1/1000 part of a milligram. The three most important weights

7

that a nurse should memorize are the microgram, the milligram and the gram. A useful tip to remember when calculating doses is that to convert grams to milligrams and milligrams to micrograms you move the decimal point *three* places.

Thus:     1·4 grams     = 1400 milligrams
          1·08 milligrams = 1080 micrograms

## METRIC VOLUMES

**Standard unit for measuring by volume: litre**
          10 millilitres = 1 centilitre
          10 centilitres = 1 decilitre
          10 decilitres = 1 litre

Only two stages are in common use, the millilitre and the litre.

**Note:** 1000 millilitres = 1 litre.

1 litre of water weighs 1 kilogram and occupies a volume of almost exactly 1000 cubic centimetres (cc or $cm^3$). Therefore 1 cubic centimetre = 1 millilitre. This fact must be noted because, although in medicine and pharmacy the millilitre is the standard unit, some prescribers still use the term 'cc'. As far as nurses are concerned they can assume that 1 ml = 1 cc.

## LINEAR MEASUREMENTS

The British system used the inch, foot and yard, with very awkward multiples such as
          12 inches  = 1 foot
          1760 yards = 1 mile

**Base unit for length: metre**

In the SI system all multiples are tens.

> 10 millimetres (mm) = 1 centimetre (cm)
>
> 100 centimetres   = 1 metre (m)
>
> 1000 metres      = 1 kilometre (km)

## UNITS OF ACTIVITY

Normally a medicine is presented as a given weight per tablets such as aspirin 300 mg, or in the case of a solution, so much weight in a given volume, e.g. morphine 10 mg in 1 ml.

For some preparations it is not possible to use weights. These are mainly antibiotics (such as penicillin) or substances extracted from animal or human tissues such as insulin or heparin.

These products have their dosages expressed as units. A prescription for insulin for instance might read:

Soluble insulin 32 units each morning.

Heparin injection 5000 units.

The range of units used varies very widely. Insulin units have 100 units per ml. Heparin units range from 1000 to 25 000 units per ml. Some antifungal drugs have their strengths measured in hundreds of thousands of units, e.g. Nystatin – 500 000 units per tablet and Nystatin 100 000 units per ml.

In order to avoid the use of a string of noughts, the term 'megaunit' is employed. 1 megaunit = 1 million units.

It must be emphasized that *each product has its own scale of units of strength*. There is no overall standard unit which applies to all preparations.

# CHAPTER ONE
## TEST YOURSELF

1. What is the name of the base unit for the amount of a substance? _____

2. What SI unit symbol is used to describe mass? _____

3. How many millilitres in 1 litre? _____

4. Convert 0·2 kg to milligrams. _____

5. If a patient requires 1 litre of intravenous fluid in 6 hours, how much should he receive every hour? _____

6. An atropine sulphate injection contains 0·4 mg in 1 ml; how many micrograms per ml ($\mu$g/ml)? _____

7. What number is $10^6$? _____

8. What percentage of a metre is a centimetre? _____

9. If a glass contains 200 ml, how many glasses would the patient have to drink to achieve 2 litre fluid intake? _____

10. What quantity does the pascal unit measure? _____

For answers see page 72.

## Chapter Two

## Interpretation of Prescription and Calculation of Doses

Normally one would expect a prescription to be a communication between doctor and pharmacist. This is not so in a hospital because there are many occasions when the pharmacist does not see the prescription and it is left to the nurse to read it. The method being adopted now by many hospitals is in line with a recommendation of a Department of Health report of January 1970. Here, a prescription sheet is used which gives instructions regarding dosage and states the precise time at which the drug is to be given. Adjoining the prescription is a space for the nurse to indicate that the drug was administered at a particular time on a given day.

With this system such phrases as 'three times a day' and 'every 6 hours', which are open to different interpretations, are no longer used. The use of Latin and Roman numerals too has disappeared, and English is used throughout.

Items dispensed for a particular patient by the hospital pharmacy will not give any instructions on the label, but will merely state the patient's name and the name of the drug and its strength. The strength on the label may not be the dose called for by the prescription so it is vital that the nurse should be able to calculate just how much to give. *Any nurse in doubt should never be afraid to admit it, and to seek advice.*

# CALCULATING THE CORRECT DOSE

## Fluid preparations taken orally

*Linctuses and elixirs and children's (paediatric) doses*
There is no difficulty here because all medicines in this group are formulated to a 5 ml dose, or multiples of 5 ml – e.g. the prescription calls for ampicillin 500 mg; the label on the container says 250 mg in 5 ml, therefore you give 2 × 5 ml. If, however, the situation were reversed and the label said 250 mg in 5 ml and you only require 125 mg, it is *not* permitted to give ½ × 5 ml by 'guessing' at half a 5 ml spoonful. The British National Formulary (BNF) states that if the dose is less than 5 ml, the pharmacy should dilute the preparation with a *suitable diluent* to bring the dose up to 5 ml. It must be emphasized that this is *not* just a question of adding water. It is the responsibility of the pharmacist. A standard 5 ml spoon should always be used.

*Adult mixures*
Here we are concerned with mixtures such as Mist. potassium citrate (commonly used to relieve cystitis). The dose called for would most likely be 10 ml and the prescription might read:

Mist. potassium citrate – 10 ml in water.

The water in this case is added *after* the dose has been poured out and the nurse is permitted to do this at the bedside at the time of administration.

**Injections**

Many injections are issued in single dose ampoules, often in several strengths. For example,

> Morphine sulphate 10 mg in 1 ml
> Morphine sulphate 15 mg in 1 ml.

In these instances there will be a sufficient range of strengths available so that it is simply a matter of choosing the ampoule which contains the correct amount. No calculations are involved.

However, the situation might arise where you require 30 mg of pethidine and you only have 50 mg per ml ampoules. In this case you apply the same method of calculation as you do for the dilution of lotions, and divide the dose required by the dose available (see page 39). For the above example this would be as follows:

$$\frac{\text{Dose required}}{\text{Dose available}} = \frac{30}{50} = \frac{3}{5} = 0.6 \text{ ml}$$

Therefore you draw up 0.6 ml from the ampoule.

Another example might be: 15 mg dose of papaveretum is required and the ampoule available contains 20 mg per ml.

$$\frac{\text{Dose required}}{\text{Dose available}} = \frac{15}{20} = \frac{3}{4} = 0.75 \text{ ml}$$

Therefore you draw up three-quarters of the 1 ml.

If however the injection is supplied in a rubber-capped vial (referred to as a 'multidose' container), the label will again state the strength as either a weight (e.g. mg) or so many units per ml. Because there are a number of doses in such a container a calculation will be necessary.

A dexamethasone injection, for instance, is issued in 2 ml vials and contains 4 mg per ml. Let us assume that the prescription calls for 6 mg dexamethasone. As there are 4 mg in 1 ml, we divide the dose required by 4:

$$\frac{6}{4} \times 1 = \frac{3}{2} = 1 \cdot 5 \text{ ml}$$

Therefore you give 1·5 ml.

Similarly a heparin injection is supplied in 5 ml vials with 5000 units per ml. Say the prescription reads heparin 10 000 units; 5000 units in 1 ml means 10 000 units in 2 ml, therefore give *2 ml*.

Injections are usually issued in strengths that fit the dose required and the answer to any calculation is seldom anything other than a whole number, as in the examples above. The exception is in paediatric doses, where calculations are commonly required.

*Use of the formula*

$$\frac{\text{Dose prescribed}}{\text{Dose available}} \times \text{volume available}$$

is often essential. An easier way to remember this formula is

$$\frac{\text{What you want}}{\text{What you have}} \times \text{amount of dilution}$$

Examples
  (a)  Dose prescribed is flucloxacillin injection 125 mg
       Dose available is flucloxacillin 250 mg in 2 ml.

$$\frac{125}{250} \times 2 = \frac{1}{2} \times 2 = \frac{2}{2} = 1 \text{ ml}$$

  (b)  Dose prescribed is diazepam 2 mg
       Dose available is diazepam 10 mg in 2 ml

$$\frac{2}{10} \times 2 = \frac{4}{10} = 0.4 \text{ ml}$$

## Doses of insulin

Accuracy of dosage is *absolutely vital* in the case of insulin injections. *An incorrect dose is liable to make a patient go into a coma.* Insulin doses are worked out individually for each patient in conjunction with his particular needs. Doses are calculated in 'units', and the insulins are now manufactured in a strength of 100 units per ml (a change which took place in the United Kingdom in 1983). The doses likely to be prescribed, however, are not multiples of 100 units. As already mentioned, doses are calculated individually for each patient and they can be anything from below 10 units to over 100 units per day. Doses such as 16, 48 or 88 units would frequently be prescribed at a diabetic clinic.

A special diabetic syringe known as BS1619/2 is used instead of an ordinary hypodermic syringe, and this has each unit marked on an 0·5 ml syringe and every alternate unit marked on a 1 ml syringe. The advantage of this syringe is that the marks are widely spaced so that an accurate dose can be drawn up.

The syringe can be and is used by all diabetics in any part of the country. This avoids confusion.

The illustrations (*Figs 1 and 2*) are actual sizes. The nurse therefore must know what she is about because she will have the task of teaching the patient.

To help the patient further when he is discharged from hospital he is given a card with all the relevant details regarding strengths of insulin to be used and how many marks on the syringe to draw up for each dose. Again, the nurse will have to explain this.

Fig. 1    Actual size insulin U100 syringes

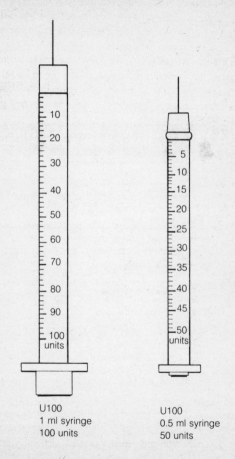

U100
1 ml syringe
100 units

U100
0.5 ml syringe
50 units

## I AM A DIABETIC ON INSULIN

Name_____

Address_____

_____

Telephone_____

If I am found ill, please give me 2 teaspoons of sugar in a small amount of water or 3 of the glucose tablets which I am carrying.
**If I fail to recover in 10 minutes, please call an ambulance (Dial 999).**
The British Diabetic Association
10 Queen Anne Street, London W1M OBD

Fig. 2(a)   Diabetic card – front

Hospital/Clinic/GP _____

Date _____

|         | Type(s) of insulin | Dose(s) |
|---------|--------------------|---------|
| Morning |                    | units   |
|         |                    | units   |
|         |                    | units   |
|         |                    | units   |
| Evening |                    | units   |
|         |                    | units   |

**ALWAYS CARRY THIS CARD WITH YOU**

Fig. 2(*b*)   Diabetic card – back

# CHAPTER TWO
## TEST YOURSELF

1. If the dose required is 500 mg, and the solution available has 50 mg per ml, how many ml should be given? _____

2. An injection contains 100 mg in 5 ml, and the dose required is 30 mg. How much should be given? _____

3. If the dose required is 35 units, and the solution available has 100 units per ml, how many ml should be given? _____

4. If the dose required is 4 mg and the solution available has 10 mg in 5 ml, how much should be given? _____

5. If the dose required is 100 $\mu$g and the solution available is 1 mg in 10 ml, how much should be given? _____

6. If the dose required is 150 mg and the solution available is 1 g in 10 ml, how much should be given? _____

7. If the dose required is 75 mg and the solution available is 250 mg in 10 ml, how much should be given? _____

8. How does an insulin syringe differ from a standard 1 ml syringe? _____

9. What is the strength of all insulin preparations? _____

10. If the dose required is 5000 and the solution contains 10 000 units per ml, how much should be given? _____

## Chapter Three

## Body Fluids – Millimoles – Physiological Saline

### FLUIDS AND ELECTROLYTES

For a normal healthy individual, that is to say a person who is neither abnormally thin nor overweight and carrying excess fat, 60% of the total body weight is fluid. This means that for a 70 kilogram (about 11 stone) man his body fluid would be approximately 42 litres (since 1 litre of water weighs 1 kg). Remember that body tissue is made up of cells which are surrounded by fluid. The fluid inside the cells is called *intracellular*, the part surrounding the cells is referred to as the *interstitial fluid* (or tissue fluid). In addition there is the enclosed circuit of the bloodstream. The fluid in the bloodstream plus the interstitial fluid make up the *extracellular fluid*. In our example the 42 litres would be distributed thus:

Intracellular fluid 28 litres (two-thirds of the total)
Extracellular fluid 14 litres (one-third of the total).

Of the 14 litres of extracellular fluid,

10·5 litres are interstitial fluid
3·5 litres are blood plasma.

The next fact to note is that body fluid is not just water

but is a solution containing a number of chemical substances (see Table 1, page 26). When a chemical such as sodium chloride (chemical symbol NaCl) is dissolved in water it becomes separated into its constituent atoms, namely sodium (Na) and chlorine (Cl). In the case of sodium chloride, nearly all the particles acquire an electric charge. The sodium becomes positively charged ($Na^+$) and the chloride takes on a negative charge ($Cl^-$). These charged particles are called *ions*. When the salt is completely dissolved, a state of *equilibrium* is reached between the dissociated ions (the $Na^+$ and $Cl^-$) and the combined constituent atoms called the *molecule* (NaCl). Thus

$$Na^+ + Cl^- \rightleftharpoons NaCl$$
(ions)       (molecule)

The charged ions are collectively known as *electrolytes*.

In the case of a substance such as dextrose ($C_6H_{12}O_6$) there is no dissociation when it is dissolved; the molecules remain unchanged. This is called a *non-electrolyte*.

Depending on the nature of the materials used, a solution can therefore contain a mixture of ions and molecules or molecules only. In a complex mixture such as blood plasma and other body fluids, all are present.

In normal health the concentration of the various particles remains constant within very narrow limits, and a balance will exist between the various ions, e.g. sodium, potassium, chloride, bicarbonate.

If in ill-health the balance is upset and there is a deficiency of one or more ions, in order to treat the patient with replacement fluid it is necessary to know 'how upset'. A sample of the patient's blood is therefore sent to the laboratory for examination. For many years it has been the practice of the pathology departments to report the results either as *milliequivalents per litre* (mEq/l), or as a *weight in volume*, usually so many mg per 100 ml. Similarly, intravenous fluids were labelled in a like manner, so solutions with ions (electrolytes) present were labelled with the milliequivalent strength and as a percentage solution, e.g. physiological saline – sodium chloride 0·9% containing 154 milliequivalents $Na^+$ per litre and 154 milliequivalents $Cl^-$ per litre. For non-electrolytes such as glucose the percentage strengths only were used.

Both methods have faults and limitations. Remember that body fluids are really chemical solutions with substances present that have an influence on (react with) one another. Both laboratory reports and the labels on the injections should therefore indicate the *reactivity* of the substances present, also what influence the level of concentration (that is, number of particles present) will have on the system as a whole. The old milliequivalent method could only be used for a limited number of ions and to report merely as the weight. It did not indicate the *number of particles* present in the system, and this is the vital factor, as the following example shows.

Imagine you have two football matches taking place, and that the total weight of each crowd is identical, at 100 000 kg. At match A you have 1000 fans each weighing 100 kg, and at match B there are 2000 fans each weighing 50 kg. The noise and discussion, the influence on the system (the football game) will be much more at match B than at match A, yet their weights are the same. It is the number of particles present which will indicate the reactivity.

The SI system is ideal for this because it can be used for

both electrolytes and non-electrolytes and will state the number of particles present in the system. Under SI units the *molar concentration* is quoted for both the laboratory reports and the labelling of intravenous fluids. This is based on the *molecular weight* of the compound. This needs further explanation.

The molecular weight of a compound is the sum of the atomic weights of its constituent elements. Water ($H_2O$) for example has a molecular weight of 18 made up of:

$$2 \text{ hydrogen atoms (atomic weight } 1) = 2$$
$$1 \text{ oxygen atom} \quad \text{(atomic weight } 16) = 16$$
$$\text{total} \quad 18$$

Similarly, the molecular weight of glucose, which has the formula $C_6H_{12}O_6$, can be calculated in the same way:

$$6 \text{ carbon atoms} \quad \text{(atomic weight } 12) = 72$$
$$12 \text{ hydrogen atoms (atomic weight } 1) = 12$$
$$6 \text{ oxygen atoms} \quad \text{(atomic weight } 16) = 96$$
$$\text{total} \quad 180$$

*The molecular weight of a substance expressed in grams is called a mole (mol)*, and a molar solution contains 1 mole per litre (mol/l) – for example, a molar solution of dextrose contains 180 grams (g/l) per litre.

The SI units system extends the term mole to apply to single ions or atoms and the ionic or atomic weight will be used for calculations. Sodium has an atomic weight of 23, therefore a molar solution of sodium ions will contain 23 grams per litre.

However, the mole is too big a unit for the convenient

measurement of body fluids, so one-thousandth of a mole is the unit used, called a *millimole (mmol)*. This is the molecular weight of a substance expressed in milligrams (one thousandth of a gram).

A bag of glucose saline labelled in SI units would have the following details:

500 ml
Glucose 4%
Sodium chloride 0·18%
Sodium chloride 1·8

| gram per litre | 30 millimole $Na^+$ per litre (mmol/l) |
| | 30 millimole $Cl^-$ per litre (mmol/l) |

Anhydrous glucose
    40·0 gram per litre     222 millimole glucose per litre (mmol/l)

Energy content of glucose 670 kJ in 1 litre (see Chapter 7 for details of energy values).

We now need to look at body fluids in a little more detail to illustrate their application. We have seen earlier (page 21) that body tissue is made up of cells and fluid, which may be either intracellular or extracellular fluid. Some of the elements present in normal health (concentrations in millimoles per litre) are as follows (see Table 1, p.26).

We can see that there are instances where there are marked differences in the concentration of some ions between the two 'compartments', most of the sodium being contained in the extracellular fluid, whereas nearly all the potassium is confined to the inside of the cells which do not contain any chloride at all.

The figures given in Table 1 are average normal values.

The actual figures will vary slightly from one individual to another, but they are always within a given range. Sodium, for instance, quoted as 142 millimoles per litre, is within the range 138 to 145.

Table 1

|  | Extracellular fluid | Intracellular fluid |
|---|---|---|
| Sodium ($Na^+$) | 142 | 8 |
| Potassium ($K^+$) | 5 | 151 |
| Calcium ($Ca^{2+}$) | 2·5 | 1 |
| Chloride ($Cl^-$) | 103 | 0 |
| Bicarbonate ($CO_3^{2-}$) | 27 | 10 |

Let us now take a specific example of a patient who gave a sample of blood examined by the hospital laboratory, and the report gave his sodium concentration as 130 millimoles per litre.

Reference to Table 1 above shows a normal sodium content as 142 millimoles per litre. This man therefore has a deficiency of 142 minus 130, i.e. 12 millimoles per litre. We have already seen that a 70 kg man has 14 litres of extracellular fluid. He would therefore need $14 \times 12 = 168$ millimoles of sodium to replace his deficiency. One litre of the intravenous fluid called physiological (previously normal) saline, which is 0·9% sodium chloride, with a concentration of 154 millimoles per litre of sodium chloride, would be adequate to treat this patient.

There is a particular reason for calling the solution of sodium chloride physiological saline: it has been shown that there is a marked difference between the compositions of the intracellular and the extracellular fluids and that the balance between the two is kept constant in normal health. The partition between these two sections (or 'compartments') of body fluid is the cell wall. Cell walls have the property of being semipermeable, and they will only allow water and certain selected materials to pass through them from one compartment into the other. This process is known as *osmosis*, and the pressure exerted by the different concentrations across the cell wall is called *osmotic pressure*. The osmotic pressure exerted by a substance in solution is dependent on the number of particles of that substance present. In the case of electrolyte solutions containing substances which dissociate almost completely into ions, the number of particles will be the same as the number of ions. The particles in a solution of a non-electrolyte (for example, dextrose or urea) will be the molecules, and the osmotic pressure created will be in direct proportion to the number of molecules present. If, therefore, the strength of the solution is doubled, the osmotic pressure will double as well.

The usual way to demonstrate osmotic pressure is to set up a simple experiment in which a sugar solution contained in a sac of parchment paper is dipped into a beaker of water. The sugar solution can be regarded as the intracellular fluid contained in a giant cell, surrounded by tissue fluid which is the beaker of water. The parchment paper (semipermeable) represents a cell wall (*Fig. 3*).

Because the sugar solution is more concentrated, water will pass through the membrane in an attempt to achieve a state of equilibrium, and the liquid in the manometer tube (usually mercury) will rise from level A to level B, showing that a pressure has developed. If you now replace the sugar

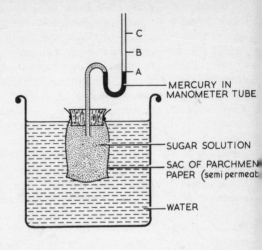

Fig. 3    Experiment set up to demonstrate osmosis

solution with one of twice the strength, the level in the manometer tube will rise twice as high as before, to C. Thus, doubling the concentration of the solution has caused the osmotic pressure to double (*Fig. 4*).

To return to the human body. Red blood cells have a peculiar biconcave shape, appearing like a disc with a depression in the middle. The outer covering of these red cells functions as a semipermeable membrane. Inside is a fluid containing free ions and, of course, the oxygen-carrying haemoglobin. Any movement of fluid and ions into and out of cells will be by osmosis, and red blood cells have an osmotic pressure just as tissue cells do. It is desirable if

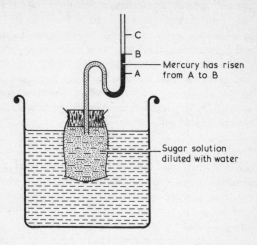

Fig. 4    Result of experiment to demonstrate osmosis

any large quantity (such as a litre) of fluid is injected into the bloodstream that the solution should have the same osmotic pressure as the red cells. Such a solution is said to be *isotonic* with blood plasma. In the case of the 0·9% sodium chloride solution used to treat the 70 kg man it is called *physiological saline*.

Let us consider what would happen if the solution were other than normal. If the solution had a higher concentration than 0·9% when injected, water would pass out of red cells into the plasma in an attempt to balance the concentration, and the cells would shrink. If the situation were reversed and the injection solution was weaker than the solution inside the red blood cells, water would pass into the more concentrated red cells in an attempt to achieve equilibrium. If this went on long enough, sufficient water would pass into the cells to swell them to a point where they would burst, releasing the red haemoglobin. This process is called *haemolysis*. Solutions stronger than isotonic are called *hypertonic* and those weaker than isotonic are called *hypotonic*. Red blood cells are sufficiently elastic to allow both hypertonic and hypotonic solutions to be given, but the strength and the rate at which they are given need careful control.

Other solutions administered intravenously are in the main given for their food value, such as glue (carbohydrate) and solutions of fats and proteins. Although, unlike electrolyte solutions, they are not ionized, some solutions such as glucose and urea do exert an osmotic pressure (see page 27) and 5% glucose is isotonic with blood. The energy value of these preparations is important and is quoted on the label.

Electrolyte solutions such as physiological saline will not mix with fat emulsions such as Intralipid, because the emulsion would break up into lumps of fat in the fluid like curdled milk. *If injected, such a solution would be dangerous.* It is now provided by the pharmacy in the form of 3-litre bags, which can be infused through a central venous catheter.

# CHAPTER THREE
## TEST YOURSELF

Complete the following:

1. Extracellular fluid is found in the tissues and in the
   _____.

2. Negatively and positively charged particles are called
   _____.

3. The molecular weight of a substance expressed in grams is called a _____.

4. The normal range for sodium levels is _____ mmol/litre.

5. Osmotic pressure is the pressure exerted by different concentrations across _____.

6. A solution containing the same osmotic pressure as the red cells is said to be _____.

7. The concentration of physiological saline is sodium chloride (NaCl) _____.

8. Sodium chloride 0·18% has _____ g/litre of sodium and chloride.

9. Solutions stronger than the solutions found in the blood are called _____.

10. What solution of glucose is the same as found in the bloodstream? _____

# Chapter Four

# pH Values

Until the 1970s is had always always been customary when testing urine to use litmus paper and report the urine as either acid or alkaline. This is still being done, but the more accurate method of testing using reagent strips is now adopted. This enables the nurse to report the 'degree' of acidity or alkalinity, and the pH value can be read off by comparing colour changes with the testing strips colour chart. In medicine, pH values are a necessary piece of information, not just for urine but with reference to many solutions. This is particularly important when 'additives' are injected into an intravenous drip fluid. Sometimes solutions have to be adjusted to a given pH value before they can be administered.

We have been seen in Chapter 3 dealing with millimoles that the composition of body fluids is kept at a constant level, and that in normal health any deviation from this level is within very narrow limits. Similarly, the degree of acidity or alkalinity of body fluids is also maintained within narrow limits, by means of a very efficient buffering system. This is known as the *acid-base balance*. Some body fluids such as blood and extracellular fluid are always *alkaline*, and others such as gastric juices and urine are always *acid*.

We noted in Chapter 3 that sodium chloride, when dissolved in water, ionized into sodium and chloride ions. It is also a fact that water ($H_2O$) ionizes very slightly into hydrogen ions ($H^+$) and hydroxyl ions ($OH^-$).

$$H_2O \rightleftharpoons H^+ + OH^-$$

Any aqueous solution therefore always contains some of these ions. Solutions which have a higher concentration of hydrogen ions over hydroxyl ions are acid in reaction and solutions with a preponderance of hydroxyl ions over hydrogen ions are alkaline.

It can be shown experimentally that the very purest of water contains equal numbers of hydrogen and hydroxyl ions. The amount is extremely small and is one ten-millionth, $\dfrac{1}{10\,000\,000}$ or 0·000 000 1 gram of hydrogen ions per litre. This water is considered *neutral* – that is, neither acid nor alkaline.

Now clearly it would be very difficult when discussing the subject to have to deal with such awkward figures as 0·000 000 1. We therefore use the indices of the SI unit system, e.g. 0·000 000 1 is written $10^{-7}$. Remember, the index figure for quantities less than one is always *one more* than the number of noughts to the right of the decimal point.

For application to the pH scale, for simplicity the index figure is used, but the (negative) minus sign is ignored. This means that for a solution of pH 6 we know that the concentration of hydrogen ions is $10^{-6}$ or 0·000 001 gram per litre.

Note that a change of one in the index figure is of course a *ten-fold* change in concentration, and a solution of pH 6 will contain ten times more hydrogen ions than that of pH 7, and is more acid. Therefore we can always say that a solution with Ph below 7 is acid, and one with pH above 7 is alkaline.

34

# CHAPTER FOUR
## TEST YOURSELF

1. What does pH measure? _____

2. Give two examples of acid body fluids. _____

3. Give two examples of alkaline body fluids. _____

4. Which ions determine the pH? _____

5. What is a neutral pH? _____

## Chapter Five

## Solutions and their Dilution

A solution can be defined as a liquid known as the *solvent* in which is dissolved another substance called the *solute*. The solute can be:

(*a*)   a solid such as salt or sugar;
(*b*)   another liquid such as glycerin;
(*c*)   a gas such as formaldehyde or ammonia.

The vast majority of solutions used in hospitals have water as the solvent, but alcohol is also used, particularly in the preparation of antiseptics. Oils, too, are used as solvents where the solute is not soluble in water. Vitamins A and D, for instance, are oil-soluble substances. Glycerin can be either a solute or a solvent.

When we describe the strength of a solution, we are in fact saying what proportion of solute is present in a given quantity of solvent. This can be expressed not only as a proportion, such as a 1 in 4 solution, but also as a *percentage*, which of course is *the amount which is present in 100 parts of solution*. Thus 1 in 4 becomes 25 in 100 or 25%. Solutions are prepared in a number of ways depending on the nature of the materials used and the type of solution required.

# WEIGHT IN VOLUME (W/V) SOLUTIONS

When a solid substance (such as common salt) is dissolved in a liquid, the usual method of preparing such a solution is to *weigh* the solute and *measure* the liquid solution in a volumetric measure. This means in effect that a 1 in 500 (w/v) solution has 1 gram of solid dissolved in water, and the whole is made up to a final volume of 500 ml. It is not 1 gram *added to* 500 ml of water and then dissolved, because the 1 gram of solid occupies a certain volume and the final solution would be more than 500 ml.

## Examples
If:
(a) *1 gram is dissolved in 1000 ml of solution*
  Expressed as a ratio, this is *1 in 1000 (w/v)*.
  Since 1000 ml contain 1 gram, 100 ml will contain 0·1 gram.
  Therefore, expressed as a percentage, this is *0.1% (w/v)*.
(b) *10 mg are dissolved in 100 ml*
  Expressed in grams, this is 0·01 g in 100 ml.
  Expressed as a percentage, this is *0·01% (w/v)*.
  Since 0·01 g are contained in 100 ml, 1 g will be contained in 10 000 ml.
  Therefore, expressed as a ratio, this is *1 in 10 000 (w/v)*.
(c) *50 μg are dissolved in 5 ml*
  By proportion, there will be 1000 μg in 100 ml.
  1000 μg = 1 mg = 0·001 g in 100 ml.
  Expressed as a percentage, this is *0·001% (w/v)*.
  Since 0·001 g are contained in 100 ml, 1 g will be contained in 100 000 ml.
  Expressed as a ratio, this is *1 in 100 000 (w/v)*.

Note that, in all the examples, whatever the unit used to express the amount by weight initially, this must be converted to grams in order to express the strength, whether as a percentage or as a proportion or ratio.

## VOLUME IN VOLUME (V/V) SOLUTIONS

With this type of solution two liquids are mixed and we simply take a measured volume of each, solute and solvent.

For example, a 25% solution (v/v) of glycerin in water would be 25 ml of glycerin and sufficient water to make up to 100 ml total. In this instance we have used ml as a unit of measurement but it could have been litres, say 25 litres of glycerin made up to 100 litres of final solution, and would still be a 25% (v/v) solution.

Now let us assume that we took 25 ml of glycerin and made up the solution to 100 litres.

> 25 ml in 100 litres
> = 25 ml in 100 000 ml (since 1 litre = 1000 ml)
> = 0·025 ml in 100 ml
> = 0·025% (v/v).

This could be calculated the other way round, thus:

> 25 ml in 100 litres
> = 0·025 litre in 100 litres
> = 0·025% (v/v).

The important thing to note here is that you must calculate the volumes in the *same* units in order to express the strength of the solution. In the above example both liquids were expressed first in ml and second in litres.

# WEIGHT IN WEIGHT (W/W)
## SOLUTIONS

It is sometimes necessary in pharmaceutical practice to weigh liquids. Strong acids when diluted are prepared by weighing both the strong acid (the solute) and the solvent, which is of course the water. Dilute hydrochloric acid (HCl) is described in the British Pharmacopoeia as containing 10·0% (w/w) HCl, and is prepared by *weighing* 10 grams of concentrated hydrochloric acid and adding it to 90 grams of water. To express the solutions as a percentage the same rule which was used for volume in volume solutions is applied. The measurements must also be calculated in the *same* units.


# DILUTION OF LOTIONS

On occasion a nurse may be called upon to prepare a weak lotion from a more concentrated solution that she has in her ward cupboard. Two rules must be used here to complete the calculation.

(*a*) Ensure that the strength required and the strength available are expressed in the *same* system before you work out the amount required. That is, the strengths must either all be expressed as proportions or all as percentages, and if necessary convert one to the other before applying the formula in (*b*).

(*b*) Divide the strength required by the strength available and multiply by the volume you are preparing. This gives the amount of concentrate you will need to make up the final solution.

$$\frac{\text{Strength required}}{\text{Strength available}} \times \text{final volume}$$

## Examples

(a) *Prepare 100 ml of a 2% solution using a concentrate of 1 in 5*
Strength required = 2%
Strength available = 1 in 5 = 20%

Therefore, $\dfrac{\text{strength required}}{\text{strength available}} \times \text{final volume}$

$$= \frac{2 \times 100}{20} = 10\,\text{ml}$$

Or, converting the other way:
Strength required = 2% = 1 in 50
Strength available = 1 in 5

Therefore, $\dfrac{\text{strength required}}{\text{strength available}} \times \text{final volume}$

$$= \frac{1}{50} \div \frac{1}{5} \times 100 = \frac{1}{50} \times \frac{5}{1} \times 100 = 10\,\text{ml}$$

*Answer*
Take 10 ml of concentrate and dilute to 100 ml with water.

(b) *Dilute a 1 in 500 solution to 1 in 4000 and prepare 800 ml*
Strength required = 1 in 4000
Strength available = 1 in 500

Therefore, $\dfrac{\text{strength required}}{\text{strength available}} \times \text{final volume}$

$$= \frac{1/4000}{1/500} \times 800 = \frac{500}{4000} \times 800 = 100\,\text{ml}.$$

*Answer*
Take 100 ml of concentrate and dilute to 800 ml with water.

(c) *Prepare 600 ml of a 1 in 3000 solution using an 0·5%*
   *concentrate*
   Strength required = 1 in 3000
   Strength available = 0·5 in 100 = 1 in 200

   Therefore, $\dfrac{\text{strength required}}{\text{strength available}} \times$ final volume

   $$= \frac{1/3000}{1/200} \times 600 = \frac{200}{3000} \times 600 = 40 \text{ ml}.$$

*Answer*
Take 40 ml and make up to 600 ml with water.

## CHAPTER FIVE
## TEST YOURSELF

1. Define a solution. _____

2. What percentage is a 1:2 solution? _____

3. What w/v solution is 5 g dissolved in 1000 ml? _____

4. If the solution is 0·05% (w/v), how much is dissolved in 100 ml? _____

5. In order to prepare 2 litres, how much solvent and solute are required for a 1 in 80 solution? _____

## Chapter Six

## Thermometers and Temperature

It must be appreciated that the temperature of an object is not a measure of the amount of heat it contains. Heat is a form of energy and is concerned with the movement of the molecules that make up the object which could be solid, liquid or gas. The greater the amount of movement of the molecules within an object the higher will be its temperature. Similarly when you apply heat to an object you increase the molecular movement which in turn makes that object hotter. If you apply a thermometer to that same object it will indicate that there has been a rise in temperature, but that is all it will do. It will not indicate the amount of heat present. In other words temperature is merely a means of comparing one situation with another.

Temperatures are useful data if you have baselines or normals to work from. Thus we know that a healthy individual has a temperature of 37°C. This is the normal, and when a nurse takes a patient's temperature she will be able to say whether the patient is hotter or cooler than normal, and no more.

The inventors of thermometers had to search for a normal when they came to calibrate their instruments. They knew that water, when cooled, would go solid and would not get any colder, and they also knew that water, when heated, would eventually reach a certain temperature and just boil away and not get any hotter. These two points were used for the lower and upper limits.

Fahrenheit was the first man to make a mercury thermometer with a proper scale. He achieved a lower temperature than that of ice by mixing salt and ice and believed that this was the lowest possible temperature attainable. He used this as his zero. He then followed an idea of Sir Isaac Newton and called body temperature 12°. Each degree he subdivided a further eight times, which meant that body temperature then read (12 × 8) 96°. When he eventually extended the scale to the boiling point of water he finished up with what we know today as the *Fahrenheit scale*. Because of these early beginnings we thus have 32°F for the freezing point of water and 212°F for the boiling point of water.

Some thirty years later Celsius, a scientist from Uppsala in Sweden, suggested a modified scale of 0° for freezing water and 100° for the boiling point of water. This of course is the *centigrade scale*, now called the *Celsius scale* in SI units.

It is in fact much more sensible than the Fahrenheit scale. We do not need 180 divisions between the freezing and the boiling points of water. Doctors and nurses are now using the Celsius scale and normal body temperature is taken as 37°C.

It should be mentioned here that the lowest theoretical temperature attainable is when all molecular movement ceases, and is recorded as 0° kelvin (K). This is one of the seven base units of SI and is used by scientists; 0°K is equivalent to minus 273 (−273) on the Celsius scale, or in everyday terms 273 degrees of frost.

Weather forecasts in the United Kingdom are issued quoting temperatures in both degrees F and C, and we are becoming familiar with temperatures in the 0° to 20°C

44

range. The clinical range however is much higher than this, and we need to know how to convert from one scale to another.

## CONVERSIONS

**To convert Fahrenheit to centigrade**
Subtract 32, multiply by 5 and divide by 9.
  e.g. Convert 50°F to centigrade.

$$50 - 32 = 18$$

$$18 \times \frac{5}{9} = 10$$

$$\therefore 50°F = 10°C$$

**To convert centigrade to Fahrenheit**
Multiply by 9, divide by 5 and add 32.
  e.g. Convert 10°C to Fahrenheit.

$$10 \times \frac{9}{5} = 18$$

$$18 + 32 = 50$$

$$\therefore 10°C = 50°F$$

Many people can remember to add or subtract 32 and can also remember to multiply by 5 and divide by 9 (or vice versa), but which combination to use for a particular conversion eludes them. If, however, you remember the above example, that *10°C is 50°F*, you can work out which way round you need the fraction. Figure 5 shows the scales compared.

| Fahrenheit | Centigrade |
|:---:|:---:|
| 110 | 43·3 |
| 109·5 | 43·1 |
| 109 | 42·8 |
| 108·5 | 42·5 |
| 108 | 42·2 |
| 107·5 | 41·9 |
| 107 | 41·7 |
| 106·5 | 41·4 |
| 106 | 41·1 |
| 105·5 | 40·8 |
| 105 | 40·6 |
| 104·5 | 40·3 |
| 104 | 40 |
| 103·5 | 39·7 |
| 103 | 39·4 |
| 102·5 | 39·2 |
| 102 | 38·9 |
| 101·5 | 38·6 |
| 101 | 38·3 |
| 100·5 | 38·1 |
| 100 | 37·8 |
| 99·5 | 37·5 |
| 99 | 37·2 |
| 98·4 | 36·9 |
| 97·8 | 36·6 |
| 80 | 26·7 |
| 78 | 25·6 |
| 76 | 24·4 |
| 74 | 23·3 |
| 72 | 22·2 |
| 70 | 21·1 |

Fig. 5   Comparative scale between Fahrenheit and centigrade.

To take a further example, that of normal body temperature, 98·4°F, and convert to the centigrade scale, we do the following:

$$98·4 - 32 = 66·4$$

$$66·4 \times \frac{5}{9} = 37$$

$$\therefore 98·4°F = 37°C$$

## CLINICAL THERMOMETERS

Apart from its relatively enormous size, there are a number of reasons why an ordinary wall or stem thermometer cannot be used in medicine. A clinical thermometer is small and is made to cover a limited range of temperatures. There are three types available but they all have one common feature.

A constriction is built into the tube containing the column of mercury so that when the instrument is removed from the patient the mercury does not run down into the bulb but stays up at whatever level was reached. A true temperature can thus be read, but it will be necessary to shake down the mercury past the constriction before taking another reading. This column of mercury is in fact of thread-like proportions and it would be difficult to see without the magnifying lens front which is built into the outer casing along the entire length of the thermometer.

### Normal range thermometers

This is the 'clinical' that nurses use every day and its scale ranges from 35° to 43°C (*Fig. 6*). Sometimes, however, it is necessary to take a patient's temperature by inserting the thermometer into the rectum. A rectal thermometer is used for this, and for no other purpose; it is identical to an

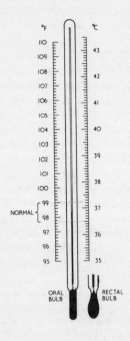

Fig. 6 A clinical thermometer, registering 35° to 43·5°C

ordinary normal range thermometer except that it has a blue-coloured bulb, merely to distinguish it from the normal type.

## Low range thermometers

It is now recognized that many patients, particularly amongst the elderly, are liable to have a condition called *hypothermia*, where body temperature is perhaps below 35°C, and the reading would be off the scale of a standard clinical thermometer. A *low reading* thermometer is available to cater for this situation. At first glance it looks like an ordinary 'clinical' and indeed it is identical except that it is designed to operate down to a temperature of 25°C.

## CHAPTER SIX
## TEST YOURSELF

1. What is boiling point on a Celsius scale? _____

2. What does the SI unit kelvin (K) measure?
   _____

3. How does a medical thermometer maintain a temperature recorded, unlike wall thermometers which alter in response to room temperature? _____

4. What is the range of a low-reading thermometer?
   _____

5. When a patient's temperature is 101°F, what is this on a Celsius scale? _____

## Chapter Seven

## Energy and Nutrition

We referred in Chapter 6 to heat being a form of energy. To be more precise this is *potential energy*, and can be described as stored energy which must be distinguished from energy of movement called *kinetic energy*. Energy is said to be indestructible, so that when you expend it in one form you change it to another. Coal contains potential energy which when burnt in a steam engine will drive that engine using kinetic energy. Chemical substances also contain potential energy and when a chemical reaction takes place, energy is released. When we eat our food we are really setting in motion a reaction similar to that of the burning coal in the engine, namely a process of oxidation. Food is, in the final analysis, a mixture of chemical substances which have potential energy. When we eat this food and digest it we turn the stored energy into both heat to keep us warm and into kinetic energy to 'drive' our bodies. For years the unit used to indicate the energy value of food was the *calorie*.

The calorie is a measure of heat and is the amount of heat required to raise the temperature of 1 gram of water from 15°C to 16°C (i.e. 1° Celsius). This was not the unit used to define the energy value of foods. For this the kilocalorie was used, which is equal to 1000 calories and was always written with a capital C.

What we really want to know is the 'mechanical energy' of

food, in other words how much work we can get from a given amount of food. The scientist Joule (born in Salford in 1818) first demonstrated the relationship between mechanical energy and energy in the form of heat. Roughly what he did was to take a vessel of water and insert in it a wooden paddle which had a number of blades projecting from a central spindle. When the paddle was rotated and the water churned up the temperature of the water went up. He was able to measure accurately the amount of energy (mechanical energy) required to turn the paddle for a given rise of temperature of the water. This became known as the mechanical equivalent of heat and the unit to measure it was called the *joule* (J); *4·18 joules are equivalent to 1 calorie* (this is of course the small calorie).

The large calorie or kilocalorie (kCal) is equivalent to 4·18 kilojoules (kJ).

$$1 \ kilocalorie \qquad = 4·18 \ kilojoules$$
$$1000 \ \text{kilocalories} = 4180 \ \text{kilojoules}$$

With SI we can extend this to a bigger unit, the *megajoule* (MJ), which is a thousand times larger than the kilojoule.

$$4180 \ \text{kilojoules} = 4·18 \ \text{megajoules}$$

In summary,

$$1 \ \text{kilocalorie (or calorie)} = 4·18 \ \text{kilojoules}$$

$$1000 \ kilocalories = 4180 \ \text{kilojoules} = 4·18 \ megajoules$$

The kilojoule and megajoule are the two standard units

under the SI system. For most practical purposes it is sufficient when working out conversions to use a figure of 4·2 (scientists use the more accurate 4·186). It will take some time for the change to become established, but it would seem sensible to use the kilojoule for the energy value of individual foods, and the megajoule for the energy content of a complete diet.

## FOOD VALUES AND ENERGY REQUIREMENTS

### Food values
The energy value of the three basic foods are as follows:

> 1 gram of protein        yields 4 calories or 17 kJ
> 1 gram of carbohydrate yields 4 calories or 16 kJ
> 1 gram of fat               yields 9 calories or 38 kJ

Table 2, pages 54–5, gives the energy content of some common foodstuffs.

We have already seen that digestion is a process of oxidation and that all foods are oxidized to carbon dioxide and water, energy being released in the process. To obtain all the avilable energy from foods, two conditions must be met: (1) the foods must be completely digested; (2) it must also be completely oxidized.

In the case of *fats*, these two conditions are met and release the full 38 kilojoules per gram. *Carbohydrates* are well digested, but many carbohydrate-containing foods also have cellulose present. This is particularly true of vegetables and the proportion varies from one produce to another. We are

## Table 2

*Energy value of some common foods*

| Foodstuff | Calories | Kilojoules |
| --- | --- | --- |
| 1 Large apple | 70 | 293 |
| 1 Large banana | 80 | 334 |
| 1 Large orange | 70 | 293 |
| 60 g Cooked prunes | 165 | 690 |
| 100 g Baked beans | 90 | 376 |
| 100 g Boiled cabbage | 8 | 34 |
| 100 g Boiled carrots | 20 | 84 |
| 30 g Fried onions | 105 | 439 |
| 100 g Boiled potatoes | 85 | 355 |
| 100 g Potato chips | 240 | 1003 |
| 25 g Potato crisps | 150 | 629 |
| 10 g Butter | 75 | 313 |
| 40 g Cheddar cheese | 160 | 669 |
| 30 g Double cream | 135 | 564 |
| 60 g Ice-cream | 100 | 418 |
| 1 Glass Cows' milk | 150 | 629 |
| 568 ml (1 pint) Cows' milk | 380 | 1588 |
| 1 Boiled egg | 80 | 334 |
| 1 Fried egg | 130 | 543 |
| 20 g Jam or marmalade | 55 | 230 |
| 30 g Milk chocolate | 170 | 710 |
| 1 Large slice white bread | 80 | 334 |
| 100 g Fruitcake | 275 | 1150 |
| 3 Cream crackers | 120 | 501 |
| 2 Digestive biscuits | 90 | 396 |

*Energy value of some common foods*

| Foodstuff | Calories | Kilojoules |
|---|---|---|
| 25 g Cornflakes | 90 | 396 |
| 150 g Fried cod | 210 | 878 |
| 100 g Steamed plaice | 90 | 396 |
| 60 g Tinned salmon | 100 | 418 |
| 60 g Fried gammon bacon | 250 | 1075 |
| 60 g Corned beef | 140 | 585 |
| 160 g Beef stew | 240 | 1003 |
| 100 g Roast leg of lamb | 230 | 961 |
| 100 g Roast leg of pork | 320 | 1338 |
| 120 g Fried pork sausages | 370 | 1546 |
| 120 g Steak and kidney pie | 360 | 1505 |
| 1 Cup of tea with milk | 20 | 84 |
| 284 ml (½ pint) Light ale | 80 | 334 |
| 1 Small sweet sherry (60 ml) | 80 | 334 |
| 2 Glasses white wine (150 ml) | 125 | 522 |
| 1 Large gin, whisky, etc. (45 ml) | 95 | 397 |

unable to digest cellulose so the food value is *nil*. It does, however, act as roughage in the alimentary canal and is of value to us in this way.

Finally, in the case of *protein*, we have to remember that the nitrogen part of the molecule is not oxidized and will not produce any energy. This part is 'lost' as urea in the urine and amounts to about 20% of the total original energy content.

**Energy requirements**

We need energy from food for four main reasons:

(a) to maintain body function, such as the action of the heart, lungs, kidneys, etc.;
(b) to keep us warm – people working in cold surroundings need more energy;
(c) for the muscular activity for work and recreation;
(d) for body growth in the case of young people.

Table 3, below, shows the energy requirements for people doing various occupations. Table 4 (pages 58–63) gives recommended daily intakes for all ages of both energy and some vitamins and minerals.

Table 3

*Average energy expended* (MJ *per day*)

| Women | | Men | |
|-------|------|-----|------|
| Bakery workers | 10·5 | Coalminers | 15·4 |
| Factory workers | 9·7 | Army cadets | 14·6 |
| University students | 9·6 | Farmers | 14·4 |
| Shop assistants | 9·4 | Building workers | 12·6 |
| Laboratory | | University students | 12·3 |
| technicians | 8·9 | Laboratory | |
| Middle-aged | | technicians | 11·9 |
| housewives | 8·7 | Office workers | 10·5 |
| Elderly housewives | 8·3 | Elderly retired | 9·7 |

Note in Table 4 the relatively high requirements for boys and girls. This extra requirement is for growth. Of the energy values quoted, 6 megajoules (about 1500 calories) are required to maintain body function and body temperature, the remainder being required for muscular activity.

How do we control our intake to suit our needs? This is quite simply done by our appetites. When we burn up lots of joules we develop bigger appetites. It sounds simple but the exact mechanism of appetite control is not known. If a person's intake of food provides more joules than are required then he/she will store the excess as fat and put on weight. A person will lose weight if he/she does not have an adequate intake of food.

Many illnesses, for a variety of reasons, will also cause a loss in weight, and these are situations when a nurse would be involved. Special diets may be ordered to meet the special needs of the patient. Each diet so ordered will supply a given number of joules. The dietician will make up the diet but nurses should know what it is all about. It has already been mentioned that 6 megajoules per day are required to maintain body functions. A diet supplying less than this will mean that the patient will call upon stored energy in the form of fat to keep him ticking over and he will lose weight. For an overweight patient a diet supplying only 3·3 megajoules per day is often prescribed.

Table 4 Recommended daily amounts of food
energy and nutrients for groups of people in the
United Kingdom (1979) (Source: DHSS)

| Age range (years) | Occupational category | Energy MJ | kcal | Protein g | Thiamin mg | Riboflavin mg |
|---|---|---|---|---|---|---|
| **Boys** | | | | | | |
| under 1 | | | | | 0·3 | 0·4 |
| 1 | | 5·0 | 1200 | 30 | 0·5 | 0·6 |
| 2 | | 5·75 | 1400 | 35 | 0·6 | 0·7 |
| 3–4 | | 6·5 | 1560 | 39 | 0·6 | 0·8 |
| 5–6 | | 7·25 | 1740 | 43 | 0·7 | 0·9 |
| 7–8 | | 8·25 | 1980 | 49 | 0·8 | 1·0 |
| 9–11 | | 9·5 | 2280 | 57 | 0·9 | 1·2 |
| 12–14 | | 11·0 | 2640 | 66 | 1·1 | 1·4 |
| 15–17 | | 12·0 | 2880 | 72 | 1·2 | 1·7 |
| **Girls** | | | | | | |
| under 1 | | | | | 0·3 | 0·4 |
| 1 | | 4·5 | 1100 | 27 | 0·4 | 0·6 |
| 2 | | 5·5 | 1300 | 32 | 0·5 | 0·7 |
| 3–4 | | 6·25 | 1500 | 37 | 0·6 | 0·8 |
| 5–6 | | 7·0 | 1680 | 42 | 0·7 | 0·9 |
| 7–8 | | 8·0 | 1900 | 47 | 0·8 | 1·0 |
| 9–11 | | 8·5 | 2050 | 51 | 0·8 | 1·2 |
| 12–14 | | 9·0 | 2150 | 53 | 0·9 | 1·4 |
| 15–17 | | 9·0 | 2150 | 53 | 0·9 | 1·7 |

| Age range (years) | Occupational category | Energy | | Protein g | Thiamin mg | Riboflavin mg |
|---|---|---|---|---|---|---|
| | | MJ | kcal | | | |
| **Men** | | | | | | |
| 18–34 | Sedentary | 10·5 | 2510 | 63 | 1·0 | 1·6 |
| | Moderately active | 12·0 | 2900 | 72 | 1·2 | 1·6 |
| | Very active | 14·0 | 3350 | 84 | 1·3 | 1·6 |
| 35–64 | Sedentary | 10·0 | 2400 | 60 | 1·0 | 1·6 |
| | Moderately active | 11·5 | 2750 | 69 | 1·1 | 1·6 |
| | Very active | 14·0 | 3350 | 84 | 1·3 | 1·6 |
| 65–74 } | Assuming a | 10·0 | 2400 | 60 | 1·0 | 1·6 |
| 75+ } | sedentary life | 9·0 | 2150 | 54 | 0·9 | 1·6 |
| **Women** | | | | | | |
| 18–54 | Most occupations | 9·0 | 2150 | 54 | 0·9 | 1·3 |
| | Very active | 10·5 | 2500 | 62 | 1·0 | 1·3 |
| 55–74 } | Assuming a | 8·0 | 1900 | 47 | 0·8 | 1·3 |
| 75+ } | sedentary life | 7·0 | 1680 | 42 | 0·7 | 1·3 |
| Pregnancy | | 10·0 | 2400 | 60 | 1·0 | 1·6 |
| Lactation | | 11·5 | 2750 | 69 | 1·1 | 1·8 |

Table 4 Recommended daily amounts of food
energy and nutrients for groups of people in the
United Kingdom (1979) (Source: DHSS)

| Age range (years) | Nicotinic acid equivalents (mg) | Total folate μg | Ascorbic acid mg |
|---|---|---|---|
| **Boys** | | | |
| under 1 | 5 | 50 | 20 |
| 1 | 7 | 100 | 20 |
| 2 | 8 | 100 | 20 |
| 3–4 | 9 | 100 | 20 |
| 5–6 | 10 | 200 | 20 |
| 7–8 | 11 | 200 | 20 |
| 9–11 | 14 | 200 | 25 |
| 12–14 | 16 | 300 | 25 |
| 15–17 | 19 | 300 | 30 |
| **Girls** | | | |
| under 1 | 5 | 50 | 20 |
| 1 | 7 | 100 | 20 |
| 2 | 8 | 100 | 20 |
| 3–4 | 9 | 100 | 20 |
| 5–6 | 10 | 200 | 20 |
| 7–8 | 11 | 200 | 20 |
| 9–11 | 14 | 300 | 25 |
| 12–14 | 16 | 300 | 25 |
| 15–17 | 19 | 300 | 30 |

| Vitamin A retinol equivalents (μg) | Vitamin D cholecalciferol (μg) | Calcium mg | Iron mg |
|---|---|---|---|
| 450 | 7·5 | 600 | 6 |
| 300 | 10 | 600 | 7 |
| 300 | 10 | 600 | 7 |
| 300 | 10 | 600 | 8 |
| 300 | | 600 | 10 |
| 400 | | 600 | 10 |
| 575 | | 700 | 12 |
| 725 | | 700 | 12 |
| 750 | | 600 | 12 |
| | | | |
| 450 | 7·5 | 600 | 6 |
| 300 | 10 | 600 | 7 |
| 300 | 10 | 600 | 7 |
| 300 | 10 | 600 | 8 |
| 300 | | 600 | 10 |
| 400 | | 600 | 10 |
| 575 | | 700 | 12 |
| 725 | | 700 | 12 |
| 750 | | 600 | 12 |

## Table 4 Recommended daily amounts of food energy and nutrients for groups of people in the United Kingdom (1979) (Source: DHSS)

| Age range (years) | Nicotinic acid equivalents (mg) | Total folate μg | Ascorbic acid mg |
|---|---|---|---|
| **Men** | | | |
| 18–34 | 18 | 300 | 30 |
| | 18 | 300 | 30 |
| | 18 | 300 | 30 |
| 35–64 | 18 | 300 | 30 |
| | 18 | 300 | 30 |
| | 18 | 300 | 30 |
| 65–74 ⎫ | 18 | 300 | 30 |
| 75+ ⎭ | 18 | 300 | 30 |
| **Women** | | | |
| 18–54 | 15 | 300 | 30 |
| | 15 | 300 | 30 |
| 55–74 ⎫ | 15 | 300 | 30 |
| 75+ ⎭ | 15 | 300 | 30 |
| Pregnancy | 18 | 500 | 60 |
| Lactation | 21 | 400 | 60 |

| Vitamin A retinol equivalents (μg) | Vitamin D cholecalciferol (μg | Calcium mg | Iron mg |
|---|---|---|---|
| 750 | | 500 | 10 |
| 750 | | 500 | 10 |
| 750 | | 500 | 10 |
| 750 | | 500 | 10 |
| 750 | | 500 | 10 |
| 750 | | 500 | 10 |
| 750 | | 500 | 10 |
| 750 | | 500 | 10 |
| | | | |
| 750 | | 500 | 12 |
| 750 | | 500 | 12 |
| 750 | | 500 | 10 |
| 750 | | 500 | 10 |
| 750 | 10 | 1200 | 13 |
| 1200 | 10 | 1200 | 15 |

# CHAPTER SEVEN
## TEST YOURSELF

Complete the following:

1. One calorie is the amount of heat required to raise
   _____ of water _____°C.

2. The unit which defines the energy value of food is called
   _____.

3. 4·18 kilojoules (kJ) = 1 _____.

4. _____ (basic food type)
   yields 9 calories per gram.

5. To maintain body function _____ calories
   per day are required.

## Chapter Eight

## Pressure Measurements

Physical pressures occur in several parts of the body, both in liquids and gases.

In both systems pressure is defined as *force* on *unit area*. Unfortunately the unit used to express these measurements is not always the same; each situation has its own unit. Blood pressure is recorded as millimetres of mercury (mmHg), and blood gases are reported in a unit called the kilopascal (kPa). We must therefore examine in more detail each situation.

### FLUID PRESSURE

Examples of fluid pressures in the body occur when you have a cavity filled with fluid. This could be urine in the bladder, cerebrospinal fluid in the central nervous system, or the more obvious one, the enclosed circuit of the blood circulation. Measurement of pressures is of considerable diagnostic value.

Imagine a metal cylinder with a base area of 10 square centimetres ($cm^2$). Now suppose we fill up the cylinder with 500 ml of water weighing 500 grams. Expressed as force per unit area we get:

$$500 \text{ grams per } 10 \text{ cm}^2$$
$$\text{i.e. } 50 \text{ grams per cm}^2$$

This is the metric unit for pressure used by physicists.

Blood vessels are of course cylindrical in shape, and unlike our imaginary metal cylinder there is no open end, and the walls of blood vessels are elastic and 'give' under the extra pressure created each time the ventricles contract.

When you take a patient's *blood pressure*, you apply pressure to the radial artery by inflating the cuff round the patient's arm. At the same time an identical pressure is applied to a column of mercury. The reading is taken in effect when the applied pressure just matches that of the artery. The height of the mercury in the tube is read off in millimetres. This is the SI unit of blood pressure recordings.

The same unit is used to record *cerebrospinal fluid (CSF) pressure*, but in this case a calibrated glass tube called a manometer tube is attached to a spinal needle by means of a short piece of nylon tubing. After the needle has been inserted into the spine, fluid is allowed to run into the tube. The height reached, which is the height above the level of the needle is recorded, again in millimetres.

## PRESSURE IN GASES

Here we are concerned with the process of breathing, which is an interchange of oxygen for carbon dioxide. In the alveoli of the lung the membrane separating the inspired air from the blood vessels is very thin, such that there is a ready interchange of these two gases. The direction of flow into or out of these blood vessels is simply determined by the pressure differential of the gases concerned, and results in oxygen going into the blood and carbon dioxide leaving the system. These pressure differentials are called *partial pressures*.

The fact that there is more than one gas present in the system (air being a mixture) does not complicate any calculations, because of the following. One of the fundamental gas laws of physics states that where you have mixed gases each behaves as though it was the only one present; and a second law says that the amount of gas dissolved in a fluid is directly proportional to the partial pressure of the gas. Therefore, in blood gas analyses, the laboratories measure the partial pressure of gases, which are recorded for oxygen as $pO_2$ and for carbon dioxide as $pCO_2$.

The unit used in the SI system is the *pascal* (Pa). A pascal is defined as the pressure exerted by a force of one 'newton' on an area measuring 1 square metre.

A *newton* (N) in turn is defined as the force required to give a mass of 1 kilogram an acceleration of 1 metre per second per second (1 m/s²).

This, you will note, consistently uses metric measurements throughout.

$$1 \text{ Pa} = 1 \text{ N/m}^2 = 1 \text{ kg/m s}^2$$

The pascal as a unit is very tiny and of no practical value in medicine. Therefore we use the *kilopascal* which is equivalent to 1000 pascal units.

$$1 \text{ kPa} = 1000 \text{ Pa}$$

For very high pressures, such as those encountered in industry, another SI unit is used. This is called the *bar*. Readers will have seen either on television or in the daily papers figures attached to each of the lines on a weather chart; these are *millibars* (*mb*).

1000 millibars = 1 bar

Some gas cylinders, such as portable oxygen cylinders used on the wards, have their contents gauges calibrated in bars. When full these cylinders have very high pressures, something of the order of 140 bars.

For those nurses familiar with the old system, a pressure conversion table is:

1 bar = 100 kPa = 14·5 lb per square inch (p.s.i.) or 750 mm of mercury (mmHg) (30 inches of mercury) on a barometer.

Turn to page 75 for revision questions on the whole book.

# Some Useful Tables

## IMPERIAL TO METRIC MEASUREMENTS IN LENGTH

| | | |
|---|---|---|
| 1 inch | = | 2·54 centimetres (cm) |
| 2 inches | = | 5·08 cm |
| 3 inches | = | 7·62 cm |
| 6 inches | = | 15·24 cm |
| 9 inches | = | 22·86 cm |
| 12 inches | = | 30·48 cm |
| 36 inches | = | 91·44 cm |

## STRENGTH OF SOLUTIONS

| | | |
|---|---|---|
| 50 $\mu$g (0·05 mg) per ml | = 0·005% | or 1 in 20 000 |
| 100 $\mu$g (0·1 mg) per ml | = 0·01% | or 1 in 10 000 |
| 400 $\mu$g (0·4 mg) per ml | = 0·04% | or 1 in 2500 |
| 500 $\mu$g (0·5 mg) per ml | = 0·05% | or 1 in 2000 |
| 1 mg per ml | = 0·1% | or 1 in 1000 |
| 4 mg per ml | = 0·4% | or 1 in 250 |
| 10 mg per ml | = 1% | or 1 in 100 |
| 20 mg per ml | = 2% | or 1 in 50 |
| 40 mg per ml | = 4% | or 1 in 25 |
| 100 mg per ml | = 10% | or 1 in 10 |

$\mu$g = micrograms
mg = milligrams

# APPROXIMATE EQUIVALENTS –
## IMPERIAL TO METRIC

**Weights**

| Imperial | Metric |
|---|---|
| 2¼ lb | 1 kg |
| 4½ lb | 2 kg |
| 6½ lb | 3 kg |
| 14 lb (1 stone) | 6·4 kg |
| 1½ stone | 9·5 kg |
| 2 stones | 12·7 kg |
| 3 stones | 19 kg |
| 4 stones | 25·4 kg |
| 8 stones | 51 kg |
| 9 stones | 57 kg |
| 10 stones | 63·5 kg |
| 11 stones | 70 kg |
| 12 stones | 76·3 kg |
| 13 stones | 82·6 kg |
| 14 stones | 89 kg |

## ELECTROLYTE (MMOL/L) AND ENERGY VALUES FOR INFUSION FLUIDS

| Solution | $Na^+$ | $K^+$ | $Ca^{2+}$ | $Cl^-$ | $HCO_3^-$ | kJ/l |
|---|---|---|---|---|---|---|
| Blood plasma | 142 | 4·5 | 2·5 | 103 | 26 | |
| Physiological saline | 150 | | | 150 | | |
| Sodium chloride 0·18% | 30 | | | 30 | | |
| Glucose 5% | | | | | | 630 |
| Glucose 5% in physiological saline | 150 | | | 150 | | 630 |
| Glucose 4·0% in sodium chloride 0·18% | 30 | | | 30 | | 630 |
| Hartmann's solution | 131 | 5 | 2 | 111 | 29 | |
| Ringer's solution | 147 | 4 | 2·2 | 156 | | |
| Sodium bicarbonate 1·26% | 150 | | | | 150 | |

# Answers to Questions
## in Chapters 1 to 7

## CHAPTER 1

1. Mole (symbol mol)
2. kg
3. 1000
4. 200 mg
5. 166 ml
6. 400 microgram/ml
7. 1 million (1 000 000)
8. 1%
9. 10
10. Pressure

## CHAPTER 2

1. 10 ml
2. 1·5 ml
3. 0·35 ml
4. 2 ml
5. 1 ml
6. 1·5 ml
7. 3 ml
8. Units are marked out – 50 on 0·5 ml syringe, alternate on 1 ml

9. 100 units/ml
10. 0·5 ml

## CHAPTER 3

1. Bloodstream
2. Ions
3. Mole
4. 138–145 mmol/l
5. The cell membrane
6. Isotonic
7. 0·9%
8. 1·8 g/l
9. Hypertonic
10. 5%

## CHAPTER 4

1. Degree of acidity or alkalinity
2. Urine, gastric juices
3. Blood, extracellular fluid, duodenal juices, bile
4. Hydrogen, hydroxyl
5. 7

## CHAPTER 5

1. Solute dissolved in a solvent liquid
2. 50%
3. 0·5% (w/v)
4. 5 g
5. 25:2000

# CHAPTER 6

1. 100°C
2. Thermodynamic (movement of molecules) temperature
3. There is a constriction in the tube containing the mercury
4. 25–40°C
5. 38·3°C

# CHAPTER 7

1. 1 g 1°C
2. Calorie (kilocalorie (kcal) – 1000 calories) N.B. Capital C is used for the large Calorie or kilocalorie (= 1000 calories)
3. Calorie
4. Fat
5. 1500

# Revision Questions

Answers are on page 78.

1. How many micrograms ($\mu$g) are there in 200 milligrams (mg)?
2. Convert 1·5 g to mg.
3. If a patient requires a total of 4 g of a substance for a course of treatment, how many days would this be using a dose regime of 250 mg four times daily?
4. Thyroxine 0·1 mg correctly written should read . . . $\mu$g.
5. How many mg per kilogram (kg)?
6. If the dose required is 1 g, and the solution available has 50 mg per ml, how many ml for the dose?
7. A patient weighs 50 kg. If the dose prescribed is 10 mg per kg and the medicine strength is 50 mg per ml, how many ml for a single dose?
8. Convert 3·5 litres to ml.
9. How many ml is 0·5 litre?
10. An injection contains 200 mg in 10 ml and the dose required is 60 mg. How many ml should be injected?
11. A corticotrophin injection has 40 units per ml, and the dose required is 100 units. How many ml should be injected?
12. Digoxin elixir is labelled 0·25 mg in 5 ml. The dose required is 2·5 $\mu$g per kg body weight and the child weighs 9·9 kg. How many ml for a dose?

13. Convert the following strengths to a percentage solution:

    (*a*) 1 in 50  (*b*) 1 in 40  (*c*) 1 in 8  (*d*) 1 in 5

14. Express these solutions as a proportion:

    (*a*) 25%  (*b*) 33⅓%  (*c*) 4%  (*d*) 12·5%

15. Express the following as percentage solutions:

    (*a*) 10 g solute dissolved, made up to 50 ml

    (*b*) 12·5 g solute dissolved, made up to 200 ml

    (*c*) 10 mg solute dissolved, made up to 25 ml

    (*d*) 200 $\mu$g dissolved, made up to 10 ml

    (*e*) 15 g dissolved, made up to 1 litre

16. You have a solution of chlorhexidine labelled as containing 50 mg in 1 ml, and require 100 ml of 1 in 2000 solution. How much of the concentrate is required?

17. Using a 20% solution of potassium permanganate, how much is required to prepare 2 litres of a 1 in 4000 solution?

18. What is the pH of the following solutions, and state whether they are acid or alkaline:

    (*a*) a solution containing 0·0001 g of hydrogen ions per litre?

    (*b*) a solution containing 0·00000001 g of hydrogen ions per litre?

19. Calculate the energy value of the following meals, giving the result in joules.

    (*a*) 1 fried egg

        1 portion (100 g) chips

        1 apple

        1 portion (60 g) ice cream

        1 glass of milk.

(*b*)  1 corned beef sandwich
(*2 slices bread*
*1 portion (10 g) butter*
*1 slice (30 g) corned beef*)
1 apple
1 portion (20 g) cheese
284 ml (½ pint) light ale.
(*c*)  1 slice of bread and butter (10 g)
1 portion (100 g) fruitcake
1 cup of tea with milk
20. How many ml in 1 fluid ounce (fl.oz)?

# Answers

1. 2000 000 $\mu$g
2. 1 500 mg
3. 4 days
4. 100 $\mu$g
5. 1 000 000
6. 20 ml
7. 10 ml
8. 3500 ml
9. 250 ml
10. 3 ml
11. 2·5 ml
12. 0·5 ml
13. (*a*) 2% (*b*) 2·5% (*c*) 12·5% (*d*) 20%
14. (*a*) 1 in 4 (*b*) 1 in 3 (*c*) 1 in 25 (*d*) 1 in 8
15. (a) 20% (b) 6·25% (c) 0·04% (d) 0·002% (e) 1·5%
16. 1 ml
17. 2·5 ml
18. (*a*) pH 4, acid (*b*) pH 8, alkaline
19. (*a*) 2886 kJ (*b*) 2235 kJ (*c*) 1817 kJ
20. 28·4 ml

*NOTES*

*NOTES*

# NOTES

# NOTES

*NOTES*

*NOTES*

*NOTES*

NOTES